Up from Agoraphobia:

How to break out of your prison of fear

by Mike McGuire

Dedication

This brief volume is dedicated to the memory of the late Dr. Arthur Hardy; and to the dozens of agoraphobics who became my friends over the years. I love you all, and wish you continued peace of mind.

Table of contents

Introduction

One evening in 1980, a friend and I were chatting on a sofa. She turned to me and said, "Someone told me something about you that I have difficulty believing."

"Oh?" I responded."What's that?"

"She said you used to be a recluse," my friend related. "I find it hard to believe you were ever a recluse."

I said, briefly, I was housebound with agoraphobia for several years, but things are fine now.

I had, indeed, come a long way from being the teen-aged boy who was confined to a small corner of his bedroom, sitting on the floor, afraid to move.

People who had helped me overcome agoraphobia had urged me to write a book about my struggle with agoraphobia. I was, they said, considered to have been one of the worst cases and had not been expected to recover, but there I was.

The book could have been of some value. At the time, there was still relatively little being written about agoraphobia, and my book would, at least, have shown other sufferers they were not alone, and that there is hope.

I passed on the idea, though, because I enjoyed my newly found freedom from fear. I was interested in continuing to move forward and not to spend a lot of time looking back.

Now, some decades later, I am writing a small volume about it. I have no explanation as to why I have decided to write it, other than I awakened from an afternoon nap and decided it would be a good idea.

In surfing the World Wide Web, I see many people with agoraphobia who feel alone, and this book is largely for them.

The pages I devote in this book to my own story are relatively brief, however, and are designed to show agoraphobics that I understand, that they are not alone, and there is hope.

The book is not a comprehensive study of agoraphobia. It is an introduction to the topic, with my ideas on how your condition can improve; with some insight on what may get in the way of recovery. Near the end of the volume, I list a number of sources I consider trustworthy for more information and help.

It is important to remember as you read these words that I am not a health care professional. What I write is based on my personal experiences. You should always consult a professional about any health issues you feel you may have.

Chapter 1 - What happened to Mike Mcguire?

The three words that best describe the Livingston, California where I grew up may be peaceful, friendly and fun.

I moved there at the age of five, in 1958. My dad had started a Southern Baptist mission there, and by 1958 the effort was successful enough to build a church on what was then called Third Street, across the street from Memorial Park.

We moved into a house about a block away on Second Street.

Life consisted of making friends, going to school, attending church, playing both sandlot and Little League baseball, taking part in scouting, collecting baseball cards, playing marbles, going to movies on weekends at Court Theater, listening to and playing rock music, and generally doing what boys enjoy doing.

There was nothing about Livingston that would obviously lead a child to develop a mental illness, but it happened to me.

My earliest memories of something beginning to go wrong with my thinking process was when I was around 10 years old. I developed a fear of being in auditoriums and other buildings at night. I imagined the lights in the buildings going out and my facing the possibility of being injured in some sort of stampede for the exits.

I don't know what brought that on. Perhaps, stories about large-city blackouts worried me, but I have no idea. The fear got in the way, however, and whenever I was in a building at night my fingers were busy scratching my thumbs to the point they developed sores, I perspired, breathed heavily and couldn't wait to get out.

In early 1965, when I was 11 years old and a sixth grader at Campus Park School, I came down with strep throat. After missing a few school days, I returned to school feeling weak, hot and generally lacking in energy. I had returned too soon, I suppose.

During that time of not feeling well physically, I was running a second lap during physical education when I suddenly felt what, in later years, I was to learn was called a severe episode of depersonalization.

I felt I was observing myself and my surroundings, outside of my body. It was like being in a dream. I was not certain whether I existed or not, and everything I saw and heard seemed unreal.

I have often thought of that moment as the moment I was simply no longer the same person anymore; and I couldn't understand why.

The episodes became more frequent and, at times, constant. Any sight or noise, any conversation, sent me into a state of numbness and unfamiliarity with my surroundings. I began to avoid everyone, not because I disliked them, but because everything "set me off."

At some point, I could no longer attend school. I was given a home teacher, but I was not well enough, not focused enough, to study; so that came to an end.

I was initially diagnosed with epilepsy and placed on medication for it, but what I had was not epilepsy.

A few months later, my dad accepted a pastorate in Modesto. I attempted to attend La Loma Junior High School in my seventh grade year, but my symptoms prevented me from attending for long, and another attempt at home teaching failed.

At the end of the school year, the Modesto School Board granted me eighth-grade standing. In retrospect, perhaps this was a mistake because I had very little instruction during my seventh grade year, and it had a particularly negative impact on my future studies in science, which had at one time been a favorite subject of mine.

In the eighth grade, I attended Modesto Christian School. It was not a hectic campus. There were 13 students in in my combined seventh-and-eighth grade class, and the teachers considered silence in the classroom as golden. I improved a great deal that year, but it was to be temporary.

During my high school freshman year, we returned to Livingston. My attendance at Livingston High School was a rarity. Two counselors served as home teachers. Bill Key was my home teacher early on, with Vince Yager taking over later.

It was during this time that my struggle with agoraphobia progressed to the point that I was confined to a small corner of my bedroom. I dreaded having to eat or use the bathroom because it meant walking a few yards, facing feelings of unreality.

They were miserable, lonely years. When my high school years were over, I earned a bachelor's degree in law through distance learning, and also studied a few courses with Southern Baptist Seminaries Extension.

Such was my existence for the next few years.

Chapter 2 - How I found out I have agoraphobia

By 1978, I had been housebound most of the time for 13 years.

If I recall, I had spent considerable time in five hospitals, being tested for every disease imaginable. The conclusion was that whatever I had was real, but was psychological rather than physical in origin.

None of the physicians uttered the word "agoraphobia," and none of the psychiatrists and psychologists I saw over the years seemed to be able to figure out what the situation was, either.

It may be that agoraphobia simply wasn't emphasized in medical school. Perhaps, it was because physicians and mental health professionals didn't run across many agoraphobics because most of us didn't venture out much.

I had no idea anyone else had what I had. Having had a religious background, there was somewhat of a belief that the whole matter was some sort of struggle between Jesus and Satan over my soul.

One Sunday night in 1978, I kicked back to watch the latest edition of "60 Minutes" on CBS.

One segment featured the work of Dr. Arthur Hardy of Menlo Park,
California, who had decided to devote his career to treating people who suffered from something called agoraphobia.

As the minutes of the segment rolled by, I saw one person after another whose situations closely paralleled mine. I was dumbfounded that, after all these years, it turned out that not only is there is a name for what I had, but there were other people who suffered from it.

A Fresno telephone number was flashed on the television screen during a commercial break for viewers wanting more information about agoraphobia; and the next day I called. On the other end of the line was a woman named Marlene Bissell, who became the first fellow agoraphobic I had ever talked to.

After psychological testing to confirm I am agoraphobic, I entered a combination group therapy/self-help program called TERRAP, an acronym for territorial apprehensiveness.

Dr. Hardy had set up several such mini-clinics throughout the United States.

The knowledge that help was finally at hand produced euphoria, but also presented a dilemma. It was great that help was available, but not so great that the help was 60 miles away.

How does an agoraphobic travel 60 miles, even for a good cause? I missed several sessions, and was allowed to go through the program a second time. The second time was a charm.

Chapter 3 - What is agoraphobia?

Agoraphobia begins with a series of panic attacks. As panic episodes become more frequent, sufferers begin to avoid situations they fear will bring on an attack, and some eventually become housebound.

Most agoraphobics do not have all the same symptoms, and we are grateful for that!

The only symptoms that fill me with dread are feelings of depersonalization and unreality, and hypoglycemic-like symptoms with shakiness and weakness.

My resting heart rate was consistently clocked above 130 beats per minute, but I don't recall being intimidated by the fast, pounding heart. I began taking beta-blockers many years ago, and a fast heart rate is largely a thing of the past.

Other agoraphobics may experience heavy sweating, cold chills, diarrhea, chest pain, stomach pain, loss of appetite, dizziness, tingly feelings in the limbs, difficulty breathing, difficulty swallowing, and a host of other symptoms.

Agoraphobics are often described as holding irrational fears of these symptoms, but we need to say a few words in our own defense.

If after years of seeing doctors and having an endless series of tests, doctors tell you the episodes are real but the cause is unknown, is your fear all that unreasonable?

Since the attacks seem to come "out of the blue," the fear they will happen again is very real and understandable.

Particularly upsetting to an agoraphobic are situations in which an escape is difficult if an attack occurs. Driving becomes difficult, especially on freeways with few exits. Crowds become a problem because there are people between you and the exit. Supermarkets and malls become difficult because of long lines and, again, people being between you and exits.

Compounding the fear of symptoms is the fear of embarrassing one's self in public. Will people think you are crazy if you make sudden exits from situations? When you are agoraphobic, can people tell simply by looking at you?

On top of symptoms and fear of what others may think, you are also hard on yourself. If you could just snap out of it, you think, or if you were a better person who had God on your side all would be well.

You miss functions important to your family and friends. You begin to feel worthless, guilty and generally depressed.

The good news is, we know more than ever what agoraphobia is and how we can enjoy improvements in our conditions.

Chapter 4 - What causes agoraphobia?

Forty years ago, agoraphobia was primarily seen as a purely psychological condition, but with the tremendous amount of research in recent decades, specialists are less certain of the causes.

Dr. Arthur Hardy of TERRAP, in the 1970s, took the position that it was primarily a psychological problem. Toward the end of his life, however, he pointed to research that suggested there were things going on in our brains that needed more exploration, and he softened his views somewhat.

"The tendency to develop panic attacks appears to be inherited," according to the National Institute of Mental Health.

Inherited, how? Is it the behavioral quirks of a parent rubbing off on a child, or is there something in the genes that cause one to be more inclined to become agoraphobic?

It is probably a little of both.

A study financed, in part, by the NIMH suggested that being bullied as a child can lead to the development of agoraphobia.

"Compared to those who went through childhood unscathed, victims had four times the prevalence of agoraphobia, generalized anxiety, and panic disorder when they became adults," the study found. "These disorders still stood even after other factors were taken into account, such as preexisting psychiatric problems or family hardships."

Another study found that people with panic disorders produce too much of a hormone called orexin.

People who produce too little orexin develop narcolepsy - a disorder in which people suddenly become drowsy and fall asleep. People who produce too much orexin have panic attacks.

"Taken together," the study concluded, "these results and other evidence suggest a critical role for an overactive orexin system in producing panic attacks."

Yet another study suggests a shortage of serotonin in the brains of agoraphobics. Serotonin is part of the chemical system in the brain that regulates emotion and emotional response.

"Brain scans revealed that a type of serotonin receptor is reduced by nearly a third in three structures straddling the center of the brain," according to the study. "The finding is the first in living humans to show that the receptor, which is pivotal to the action of widely prescribed anti-anxiety medications, may be abnormal in the disorder, and may help to explain how genes might influence vulnerability."

My layperson's opinion is that both some form of psychotherapy and some type of medication are necessary, but I am not a doctor. Listen to your doctor.

Over the decades, I was prescribed more medications than I can remember in an effort to control my agoraphobia.

There is no such thing as a drug that will cure agoraphobia, but there are medications that can take the edge off your panic to enable you to function and begin to think more clearly about how you react to life's events.

No two people are alike. Only one medication has succeeded in taking the edge off my condition. Without diazepam (Valium), recovery is much more difficult for me.

Valium, obviously, isn't for everyone. One drawback is you can become addicted to it. If you take too much of it, you may pass out and even die.

The biggest danger I have had with diazepam is the temptation to rely on it to remove causes of anxiety. Diazepam doesn't do that. If you rely too heavily on diazepam, you will now have two problems - agoraphobia and drug addiction.

I also take fluoxetine (Prozac). The stated purpose of Prozac is to have a positive impact on chemicals in the brain that may become unbalanced and cause panic.

For me, the jury is out on Prozac. I can report I don't feel worse after taking it for quite some time, but I am not convinced it has improved my situation, either.

Now that we've touched briefly on some of the possible causes of agoraphobia, let's move on to some chapters about how agoraphobics need to change the way we think.

Chapter 5 - New ways of thinking

It goes without saying - but I am going to say it, anyway - that it is impossible for a person to be anxious and relaxed at the same time.

Since the goal is to feel relaxed and at peace, the work is to develop a new way of thinking about yourself and your surroundings. Your emotions are the result of your way of thinking, behaving and reacting internally to your surroundings.

Before you can begin to think straight, you need to not only learn but become good at practicing relaxation techniques.

There are many good books available on relaxation techniques. A search on Amazon.com will turn up many volumes that you can read and try.

Not every relaxation technique is workable for everyone. When I first began learning relaxation techniques, I was somewhat confused by suggestions that I imagine being somewhere peaceful as I began my relaxation exercises. This sometimes included a suggestion that I picture myself at a beach. Well, folks, people with severe cases of agoraphobia don't go to the beach.

It is important for you to find a relaxation routine that is right for you. Checking a few books to examine various techniques is one way, as I mentioned. Asking your doctor for advice is another way.

The technique that has worked for me is progressive relaxation through the tensing of muscles, followed by letting them go.

I begin at my feet and go to the top of my head. I first tense the muscles as tightly as I can for as long as I can and then allow them to go limp.

I move on up, tensing any muscle I can find and then letting go.

I have gotten good enough at it that I have learned how to let go of anxiety rather quickly by zeroing in on muscle groups that provide the most relief.

In many office-type situations, seated at my desk, I would arch my back, tighten my back muscles as hard as I could and then let go. I would immediately sigh and feel better. It is a technique I still used. It can be used in any position - standing, sitting, reclining.

Whatever method you choose, it is important that you use it regularly. By decreasing muscle tension, you will free your mind for more pleasant and more logical thoughts. With time, you will be surprised at how much more pleasant you can feel after a severe bout of anxiety.

Chapter 6 - That's funny; you don't look nervous

As I mentioned in an earlier chapter, I spent my share of time going to psychiatrists who were of little value. I'll give them the benefit of the doubt, though, because there was a time when not much thought was given to agoraphobia.

At one session, I explained my life to a psychiatrist - the constant anxiety, frequent episodes of sheer panic, and the rest of the story.

His reaction to my story? He looked at me in the noncommittal, half-bored way psychiatrists tend to look and said, simply, "You don't look nervous to me."

One of agoraphobics' chief fears is people can tell by looking at us how we feel inside; and that people will dismiss us as weird.

But, whether it is healthy or not, agoraphobics have a natural talent at masking our feelings.

When I attended TERRAP sessions, a friend of mine and I had a friendly wager. Agoraphobics arrived at sessions with a spouse or some other support person. When a new agoraphobic would join the group, we would place a bet on which of the two was agoraphobic.

In every case, one person would walk in looking anxious and jittery; and the person he or she was with would be all smiles, looking like the most-confident person imaginable.

Initially, we always assumed the poor, nervous-looking being was the agoraphobic; and we were always wrong. The agoraphobic was always the charming one who appeared not to have a care in the world.

Most agoraphobics are charming by nature. Many of my acquaintances might be in the mood to argue that point, but some of my elementary school teachers went out of their way to write notes on my report cards about how charming I am. So there.

Agoraphobics tend to want the world to be a charming place, with people treating each other well and everything going along smoothly. Perhaps, we believe that if we are friendly, everyone else will be friendly, too, and we will have Heaven on earth.
We are people-pleasers. We will yield a little bit too much in the interests of enjoying a more peaceful inner and outer world.

This results in our being walked on, to some degree, because not everyone shares our vision of harmony.

This frustrates us, angers us, and generally leads to more anxiety over our surroundings.

So, one of the first steps an agoraphobic must take is to learn we have the right to breathe air, too. We have the right to say what type of behavior we expect from others. We have the right not to be taken advantage of.

It takes practice to say what you expect; but the more you do it the easier it becomes.

You don't have to be aggressive, just assertive. If you don't want someone to treat you in a certain way - to say certain types of things to you, just say so.

There are some wonderful books available on assertiveness training. A search on Amazon.com will turn up some good books for you to examine.

Chapter 7 - Walking is the best exercise

During my late teens and early 20s, I exercised daily using the Royal Canadian Air Force exercise as my guide.

I built up a few muscles, particularly in my legs. I could run in place at a brisk speed for 10 minutes or so.

While this was good for my cardiovascular system and gave me a few leg muscles I could be proud of, running in place won't help you recover from agoraphobia.

Getting in the best shape you can, physically, will help you overcome agoraphobia, but the exercise you get should be related to what you need to do to get better.

Doing 30 sit-ups every morning is a commendable goal, but once you've reached it, your agoraphobia is as bad as it was.

The key is to combine physical exercise with getting you out of the house. To this end, taking walks is your best bet.

If you are housebound, your reaction will be something along the line of "easier said than done," and you are right if you expect to win the battle in one day.

The task is to build yourself up emotionally as you build yourself up physically, and you can start wherever you are today.

To use a extreme example, let's say you are as housebound as I was during the days when I was confined to a small corner of my bedroom. How would someone with agoraphobia that severe get to where he or she could take leisurely strolls around the neighborhood?

You would begin my standing up. Once you have done that, you have met your immediate goal. When that becomes easy enough, perhaps you walk to your bedroom door, open it and stand there until you feel uncomfortable.

When that becomes easy or boring, you can walk to the front door of your house, keep the door closed and just stand near the door.

The next step would be to walk to the front door, open it and stand there gazing at the outside for as long as your comfortable.

Perhaps, the next trip would involve opening the door and standing on the porch for a few minutes; then later sitting on the lawn.

This will sound silly to many people, but agoraphobics get it. By gradually extending your boundaries, you will eventually win. Sit on the lawn, then walk to the edge of your yard, then walk across the street and back, and gradually increase the distance from home that is comfortable to you.

It doesn't matter how long it takes you to get to where you can comfortably enjoy yourself by taking walks. If it takes a week, fine. If it takes a month, fine. If it takes longer, fine. The important thing is you will be making progress. Slow progress is more satisfying than none at all.

If you are a "standard agoraphobic," you will be self-conscious, convinced that all eyes are on you and that people think you're weird.

People have their own lives they are concerned about. Most people are not going to be wrapped up in your taking a walk. If they are, for some reason, well . . . screw 'em. You have a right to breathe air, too.

Chapter 8 - Getting back in the driver's seat

Since it is an agoraphobic's goal to get out and do things, we started our discussion in the last chapter with walking. Now, we turn to what - for some - will be the scarier topic of getting back in your car and driving.

Perhaps, the best way to approach the topic is to simply tell you how I did it.

In my early 20s, I managed to get a driver's license on the fifth try; but I was not yet a recovering agoraphobic - I still hadn't heard the word - and after I got my license, that was the end of my driving for a long while.

Once I began getting relaxation techniques under my belt, I decided it was time to drive.

How did I begin? Much like a recovering agoraphobic gets used to walking around like a free person. I did it slowly.

I started by simply walking to my car, opening the door and getting behind the wheel. I didn't put the key in the ignition. I just sat there, getting accustomed to the feel of the car.

When that became boring, I began walking to the car, opening the door, sitting behind the wheel and placing the key in the ignition, but not starting the car.

Then came the usual routine, but this time starting the car and just sitting there.

When I could do that comfortably, I backed up the car up a few yards and then drove it back a few yards.

Then, I backed out of the driveway and drove back into it. After that became comfortable, I drove around the block.

Anyway, I think you get the routine. I worked up to it very gradually.

When I recovered enough, you couldn't keep me home. My mother drove to the TERRAP sessions, and I drove the 60 miles back.

Ultimately, I was driving by myself anywhere there was a road. I drove up and down freeways, went to movies in other cities, ate wherever I saw a cafe, haunted bookstores and record shops, visited newly found friends and, after everyone else in the world went to bed, I drove along country roads, more freeways, visited small towns for no other reason than they were there, and generally had fun with my newly found freedom from fear.

On average, I was home about three or four hours per day. I don't recommend that, at all, by the way because there is a such a thing as burning a candle at both ends.

You, too, can have more freedom and go where you please. Again, it doesn't matter how long it takes. Slow progress is better than no progress. Don't become impatient with yourself - impatience is simply a form of anxiety and emotional distress. Respect yourself, do your relaxation exercises and move at your own pace.

Chapter 9 - Agoraphobia and demon possession

Most Americans profess to be both religious and believe in the existence of Satan. Fortunately, most Americans don't translate their faith into a belief that mental and emotional maladies are either punishment from God or curses from Satan.

There is a minority within Christianity, however, who look upon fear as something to be cast out through supernatural means; and it may be you either live among them or will run into them.

I live in the San Joaquin Valley of California. If California has a Bible Belt, this is it. Being from a religious family, I am well aware of religious theories about illness, although members of my family - most of whom were Southern Baptists - don't place much emphasis on demons.

Many mainstream, conservative Christians, however, still have faulty views of illness.

During my early days of recovery, I purchased a handheld GSR device. "GSR" is an acronym for galvanized skin response. Essentially, the device measured perspiration on my skin and measured levels of anxiety that way. The higher the anxiety, the higher the tone the GSR device emitted, and the calmer I got, the lower the tone got.

I explained how it worked to a Christian woman, a Southern Baptist, and when I finished showing her how it worked, she paused and said, simply, "Oh, I believe biofeedback is of the devil."

My reaction was to simply look at her. I was dumbfounded. The woman had six years of college, in secular institutions, and yet she believed the devil was behind biofeedback.

In another encounter with Southern Baptists, the local pastor stopped by one day, accompanied by an evangelist. The church was about to have a series of revival meetings and it was explained that now that I was well enough to be out and about, I was well enough to attend revival meetings.

Having read my share of books on assertiveness training, I decided not to get into a long, philosophical discussion with the fellows and said, calmly, "I understand how you feel, but I am not interested."

The pastor responded that God could very well take away my ability to write if I didn't start going back to church.

I found if absurd that God would turn me into an illiterate if I didn't show up at his church, sit in a pew and listen to him mispronounce Deuteronomy, but I wasn't interested in a debate.

"I understand how you feel," I repeated, "but I'm not interested."

A couple more threats about what God might to do me followed, and I repeated my broken-record response. They gave up, went away, and never bothered me about their religion again.

Humanity has a long history of looking upon natural phenomena as supernatural, and centuries have been devoted to trying to pray away hurricanes, praying for rain, praying for warmer days, praying for cooler days, praying for salvation from earthquakes and floods, and so on.

Epilepsy was once seen, depending upon which culture you grew up in, as either a gift from the gods or curse from the devils. Epileptics, in many Western cultures, were seen as demon possessed and prayers for deliverance were offered for them.

Today, we know that epilepsy has nothing to do with gods or devils, but it is a disorder of the central nervous system. It's natural, not supernatural.

People with schizophrenia suffered a similar attitude from many religious people. It, too, was considered to be either demon possession or oppression by demons. Today, we know schizophrenia is a brain disorder, and the effectiveness of medication has replaced the ineffectiveness of prayer.

Religious spokespeople should be taken seriously when they discuss physical and mental ailments only if they are educated to do so. Most are not, and the best approach to dealing with people who want you to find supernatural solutions to your natural problems is to simply say, with me, "I understand how you feel, but I am not interested.

Chapter 10 - Resources for agoraphobics

Thank you for downloading and reading this booklet. My goal is to help you on your road to recovery from agoraphobia and panic disorders.

I have compiled a list of additional resources that will be helpful to you as you begin or continue your journey to freedom from fear.

The late Dr. Arthur Hardy, the pioneer in modern research into agoraphobia and founder and TERRAP, was also the first person to lead the Phobia Society of America.

In recent years, the PSA changed its name to the Anxiety and Depression Association of America.

Its website offers extension information about agoraphobia and panic disorders, publishes an e-newsletter, has an extensive library of recommended self-help books, and maintains a database of therapists throughout the United States who are trained to help people with agoraphobia.

In addition to the ADAA, there are two books I recommend that I am confident will lead to to your enjoying very satisfying improvements in your condition.

- "When Panic Attacks: The New, Drug-Free Anxiety Therapy That Can Change Your Life," by David D. Burns, MD.

- "The Anxiety and and Phobia Workbook" by Edward J. Bourne.

There are many books on the market, many of them helpful and others not. I believe these two are the volumes that will not only get you started on your way to recovery, but help you find ways to remain free from fear.

Appendix A - NIMH on panic disorder and agoraphobia

(Following is information about agoraphobia, as provided by the National Institute of Mental Health.)

What is Panic Disorder?

People with panic disorder have sudden and repeated attacks of fear that last for several minutes. Sometimes symptoms may last longer. These are called panic attacks. Panic attacks are characterized by a fear of disaster or of losing control even when there is no real danger. A person may also have a strong physical reaction during a panic attack. It may feel like having a heart attack. Panic attacks can occur at any time, and many people with panic disorder worry about and dread the possibility of having another attack.

A person with panic disorder may become discouraged and feel ashamed because he or she cannot carry out normal routines like going to the grocery store or driving. Having panic disorder can also interfere with school or work.

Causes

Panic disorder sometimes runs in families, but no one knows for sure why some people have it while others don't. Researchers have found that several parts of the brain are involved in fear and anxiety. By learning more about fear and anxiety in the brain, scientists may be able to create better treatments. Researchers are also looking for ways in which stress and environmental factors may play a role.

Signs & Symptoms

People with panic disorder may have:

- Sudden and repeated attacks of fear
- A feeling of being out of control during a panic attack
- An intense worry about when the next attack will happen
- A fear or avoidance of places where panic attacks have occurred in the past
- Physical symptoms during an attack, such as a pounding or racing heart, sweating, breathing problems, weakness or dizziness, feeling hot or a cold chill, tingly or numb hands, chest pain, or stomach pain.

Who Is At Risk?

Panic disorder affects about 6 million American adults and is twice as common in women as men. Panic attacks often begin in late adolescence or early adulthood, but not everyone who experiences panic attacks will develop panic disorder. Many people have just one attack and never have another. The tendency to develop panic attacks appears to be inherited.

Diagnosis

Panic attacks can occur at any time, even during sleep. An attack usually peaks within 10 minutes, but some symptoms may last much longer.

People who have full-blown, repeated panic attacks can become very disabled by their condition and should seek treatment before they start to avoid places or situations where panic attacks have occurred. For example, if a panic attack happened in an elevator, someone with panic disorder may develop a fear of elevators that could affect the choice of a job or an apartment, and restrict where that person can seek medical attention or enjoy entertainment.

Some people's lives become so restricted that they avoid normal activities, such as grocery shopping or driving. About one-third become housebound or are able to confront a feared situation only when accompanied by a spouse or other trusted person. When the condition progresses this far, it is called agoraphobia, or fear of open spaces.

Early treatment can often prevent agoraphobia, but people with panic disorder may sometimes go from doctor to doctor for years and visit the emergency room repeatedly before someone correctly diagnoses their condition. This is unfortunate, because panic disorder is one of the most treatable of all the anxiety disorders, responding in most cases to certain kinds of medication or certain kinds of cognitive psychotherapy, which help change thinking patterns that lead to fear and anxiety.

Panic disorder is often accompanied by other serious problems, such as depression, drug abuse, or alcoholism.These conditions need to be treated separately. Symptoms of depression include feelings of sadness or hopelessness, changes in appetite or sleep patterns, low energy, and difficulty concentrating. Most people with depression can be effectively treated with antidepressant medications, certain types of psychotherapy, or a combination of the two.

First, talk to your doctor about your symptoms. Your doctor should do an exam to make sure that another physical problem isn't causing the symptoms. The doctor may refer you to a mental health specialist.

Treatments

Panic disorder is generally treated with psychotherapy, medication, or both.

Psychotherapy. A type of psychotherapy called cognitive behavior therapy is especially useful for treating panic disorder. It teaches a person different ways of thinking, behaving, and reacting to situations that help him or her feel less anxious and fearful.

Medication. Doctors also may prescribe medication to help treat panic disorder. The most commonly prescribed medications for panic disorder are anti-anxiety medications and antidepressants. Anti-anxiety medications are powerful and there are different types. Many types begin working right away, but they generally should not be taken for long periods.

Antidepressants are used to treat depression, but they also are helpful for panic disorder. They may take several weeks to start working. Some of these medications may cause side effects such as headache, nausea, or difficulty sleeping. These side effects are usually not a problem for most people, especially if the dose starts off low and is increased slowly over time. Talk to your doctor about any side effects you may have.

It's important to know that although antidepressants can be safe and effective for many people, they may be risky for some, especially children, teens, and young adults. A "black box"—the most serious type of warning that a prescription drug can have—has been added to the labels of antidepressant medications. These labels warn people that antidepressants may cause some people to have suicidal thoughts or make suicide attempts. Anyone taking antidepressants should be monitored closely, especially when they first start treatment with medications.

Another type of medication called beta-blockers can help control some of the physical symptoms of panic disorder such as excessive sweating, a pounding heart, or dizziness. Although beta blockers are not commonly prescribed, they may be helpful in certain situations that bring on a panic attack.

Some people do better with cognitive behavior therapy, while others do better with medication. Still others do best with a combination of the two. Talk with your doctor about the best treatment for you.

Living With

"One day, without any warning or reason, I felt terrified. I was so afraid, I thought I was going to die. My heart was pounding and my head was spinning. I would get these feelings every couple of weeks. I thought I was losing my mind."

"The more attacks I had, the more afraid I got. I was always living in fear. I didn't know when I might have another attack. I became so afraid that I didn't want to leave my house."

Appendix B - Childhood Bullying Linked to Adult Psychiatric Disorders

Feb 18, 2014

By Chelsea Perugini, U.S. Department of Health and Human Services

This blog post originally appeared on StopBullying.gov

Duke University professors published research that shows the degree to which bullying can affect someone's mental health.

Authors Copeland, Wolke, Angold and Costello discovered that victims of childhood bullying have a higher risk of developing mental health problems later in life. The study followed more than 1,000 youth, starting at the ages of 9, 11 and 13. The youth were interviewed each year until they turned 16. Follow-up interviews were then conducted into adulthood.

Results of the study showed bullying elevated the rate of mental health problems. Some of the key findings were:

Youth who were victims of bullying had a higher chance of having agoraphobia, anxiety and panic disorders.

Youth who bullied were at risk for antisocial personality disorder.

Youth who bullied who were also victims of bullying were at a higher risk for adult depression and panic disorder. For this group, there was an increased risk for agoraphobia in females and suicidality in males.

The link between bullying and mental illness is very real. This research brief only scratches the surface of this issue, and is not a synthesis of all mental health and bullying research.

Bullying can have many different effects.

Bullying is a serious problem for all involved and can have a lasting impact on someone's entire life—but it doesn't have to. You can help youth heal from the harmful effects of bullying.

"My friend saw how afraid I was and told me to call my doctor for help. My doctor told me I was physically healthy but that I have panic disorder. My doctor gave me medicine that helps me feel less afraid. I've also been working with a counselor learning ways to cope with my fear. I had to work hard, but after a few months of medicine and therapy, I'm starting to feel like myself again."

About the author

Mike McGuire is a freelance writer who lives in California with his wife, Susan. They have two grown daughters, ReJon and Kisha. Mike can be contacted by email at michaelm494@gmail.com.

Mike has worked as the editor of the Livingston (Calif.) Chronicle, and has also worked for AOL, Intel, PC World, Charles Schwab and other companies.